Adjustment Cord Theory

AF212718

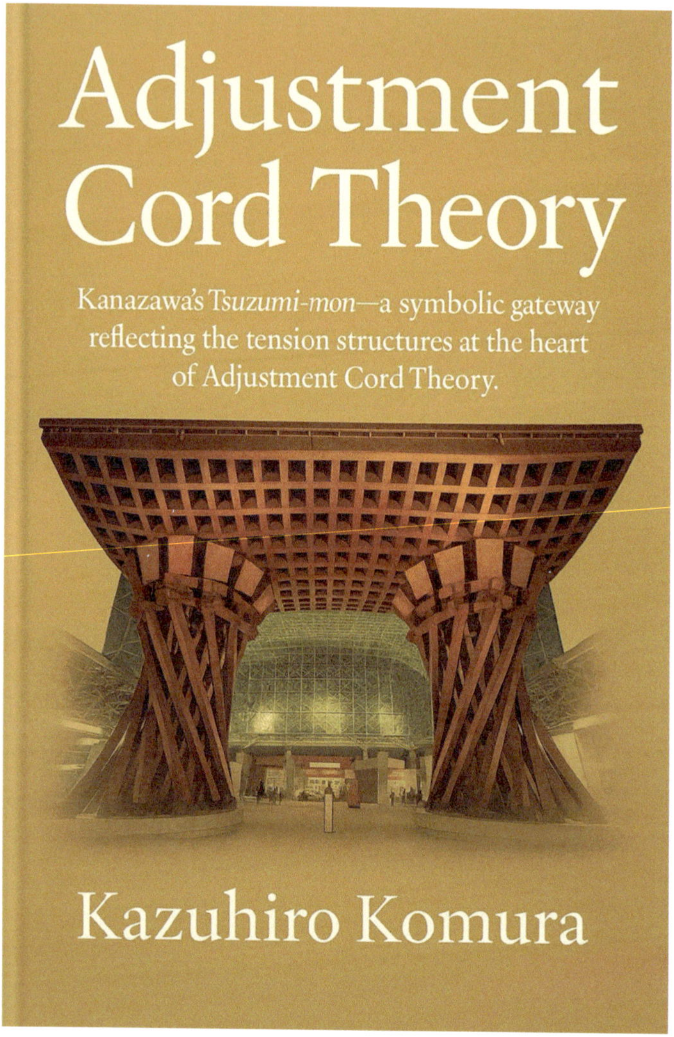

Image credit: Photograph courtesy of the City of Kanazawa

Kazuhiro Komura

Adjustment Cord Theory

Untangling Complex Disease Networks

Springer

Kazuhiro Komura
Department of Dermatology
Kanazawa Red Cross Hospital,
Japanese Red Cross Society
Kanazawa, Ishikawa, Japan

ISBN 978-981-95-7644-9 ISBN 978-981-95-7645-6 (eBook)
https://doi.org/10.1007/978-981-95-7645-6

© The Editor(s) (if applicable) and The Author(s), under exclusive license to Springer Nature Singapore Pte Ltd. 2026

This work is subject to copyright. All rights are solely and exclusively licensed by the Publisher, whether the whole or part of the material is concerned, specifically the rights of translation, reprinting, reuse of illustrations, recitation, broadcasting, reproduction on microfilms or in any other physical way, and transmission or information storage and retrieval, electronic adaptation, computer software, or by similar or dissimilar methodology now known or hereafter developed.
The use of general descriptive names, registered names, trademarks, service marks, etc. in this publication does not imply, even in the absence of a specific statement, that such names are exempt from the relevant protective laws and regulations and therefore free for general use.
The publisher, the authors and the editors are safe to assume that the advice and information in this book are believed to be true and accurate at the date of publication. Neither the publisher nor the authors or the editors give a warranty, expressed or implied, with respect to the material contained herein or for any errors or omissions that may have been made. The publisher remains neutral with regard to jurisdictional claims in published maps and institutional affiliations.

This Springer imprint is published by the registered company Springer Nature Singapore Pte Ltd.
The registered company address is: 152 Beach Road, #21-01/04 Gateway East, Singapore 189721, Singapore

If disposing of this product, please recycle the paper.

Preface

Interventions rarely fail because we lack detail. They fail because detail does not always tell us where to act.

In many complex diseases, we know an extraordinary amount. We can describe molecular interactions, cellular behaviors, and network structures with increasing precision. Yet when intervention is attempted, outcomes remain inconsistent. Effects fade, shift, or reverse. What appeared central proves bypassable. What seemed decisive turns out to be optional.

This book begins from that discomfort.

Rather than asking what drives disease, it asks where disease is structurally constrained. Rather than seeking dominant components, it focuses on passages that cannot be avoided when systems adapt. These passages—referred to here as *adjustment cords*—are not always visible, stable, or powerful. Their importance emerges only when alternatives narrow and tension is forced to converge.

The perspective developed in this book does not promise simplification. Complexity is not treated as an obstacle to be eliminated, but as a condition to be designed within. The aim is not to replace mechanistic understanding, but to orient it—to distinguish what is prominent from what is necessary.

Adjustment Cord Theory is presented as a framework rather than a solution. It offers no lists of targets, no universal algorithms, and no disease-specific prescriptions. What it offers instead is a way of reasoning about why intervention so often misses its mark, and how alignment with structural necessity might alter that trajectory.

The chapters that follow proceed deliberately. Early sections describe patterns without justification. Later chapters supply structure, dynamics, and principles of intervention. The theory is allowed to unfold gradually, resisting premature closure.

This book is written for readers who sense that something essential is being overlooked—not because it is hidden, but because it is quiet. What follows is an attempt to give that quiet structure a language.

Kanazawa, Ishikawa, Japan Kazuhiro Komura

Contents

Chapter 1
Why Complex Diseases Resist Simplification

1.1 The Persistent Difficulty of Explaining Complex Disease

Despite remarkable advances in molecular biology, medicine continues to struggle with diseases whose behavior remains difficult to anticipate and difficult to influence. This difficulty is familiar to many researchers and clinicians, not as a lack of information, but as a persistent sense that something essential is being missed. In such diseases, detailed molecular knowledge has accumulated at an unprecedented rate. Gene expression profiles, signaling cascades, cellular interactions, and environmental influences are described with increasing precision. Yet this precision has not translated proportionally into explanatory clarity or therapeutic predictability.

This gap is often attributed to incomplete data, insufficient resolution, or technical limitations. While these factors play a role, they do not fully account for the persistence of unpredictability. Even in settings where data are abundant and mechanisms are well characterized, intervention frequently produces outcomes that are inconsistent, transient, or counterintuitive.

© The Author(s), under exclusive license to Springer Nature Singapore Pte Ltd. 2026
K. Komura, *Adjustment Cord Theory*,
https://doi.org/10.1007/978-981-95-7645-6_1

The difficulty, therefore, is not simply a lack of information. It reflects a deeper mismatch between how complex disease systems are organized and how they are commonly interpreted. The discrepancy has been widely recognized in the context of network medicine, where disease is understood not as the failure of isolated components but as a perturbation of interconnected systems [1].

1.2 Heterogeneity as Structure, Not Noise

Clinical heterogeneity is often treated as an obstacle to be overcome. Patients are stratified, outliers are excluded, and variability is reduced in order to reveal underlying regularities. While such approaches are methodologically useful, they implicitly assume that heterogeneity is noise obscuring a more fundamental uniformity. Concerns regarding the limitations of conventional disease classification in the face of pervasive heterogeneity have also been articulated in postgenomic frameworks of disease taxonomy [2].

This assumption is increasingly difficult to sustain. Variability in disease expression, progression, and treatment response is not random. It is patterned, persistent, and often reproducible across cohorts. Rather than disappearing with improved measurement, heterogeneity frequently becomes more pronounced.

Adjustment Cord Theory begins from a different premise: heterogeneity is not an artifact of incomplete knowledge, but a manifestation of structure. Complex disease systems do not converge toward a single optimal state. They maintain multiple configurations under constraint, each capable of producing similar outward appearances.

From this perspective, variability is not a failure of classification. It is a property of how tension is distributed and constrained within the system. Understanding disease therefore requires attention not only to what is present, but to how alternatives remain available or become restricted.

1.3 Why Intervention Points Remain Elusive

If heterogeneity reflects structure, the persistent difficulty of identifying reliable intervention points becomes more comprehensible. Conventional strategies often focus on elements that are prominent, active, or statistically associated with disease outcomes. Such elements provide intuitive targets, yet acting them frequently yields limited or inconsistent benefit.

This pattern has led to cycles of optimism and disappointment. Promising targets demonstrate initial efficacy, followed by adaptation, compensation, or relapse. Escalation of intensity may prolong response without altering long-term trajectories. In other cases, intervention produces effects that appear paradoxical or contradictory to mechanistic expectation.

These outcomes are commonly interpreted as resistance, redundancy, or system complexity beyond practical control. Adjustment Cord Theory approaches them differently. It suggests that intervention fails not because systems are unknowable, but because action is often applied at points of visibility rather than at points of necessity.

Intervention points remain elusive because they are not defined by magnitude or prominence. They are defined by constraint. Without a framework capable of distinguishing between these properties, even well-supported interventions may be structurally misaligned. From a systems perspective, such behavior is consistent with biological robustness, whereby systems preserve function through redundancy and temporal adaptive reconfiguration despite perturbation [3].

1.4 Scope and Intent of This Book

This book proposes Adjustment Cord Theory as a framework for reasoning about complex disease systems under constraint. It does not aim to replace existing mechanistic explanations, nor does it seek to provide disease-specific prescriptions.

Instead, the theory focuses on identifying structurally imposed passages through which tension must pass in order for a system to maintain or transition between configurations. These passages, referred to as adjustment cords, are not always visible, dominant, or stable. Their relevance emerges under conditions of constraint, perturbation, and temporal change.

The chapters that follow develop this framework progressively. Early sections introduce conceptual foundations and morphological patterns without attempting full justification. Subsequent chapters translate these patterns into structural analysis, dynamics, and principles of intervention. Disease-specific detail is intentionally minimized in order to preserve generality and transferability.

Equally important is what this book does not attempt. It does not offer algorithms for identifying adjustment cords, nor does it provide exhaustive reviews of disease mechanisms. These absences are deliberate. Adjustment Cord Theory is designed to orient inquiry rather than to close it.

The aim is not to simplify complexity, but to design within it.

References

1. Barabási A-L, Oltvai ZN. Network biology: understanding the cell's functional organization. Nat Rev Genet. 2004;5:101–13.
2. Loscalzo J, Kohane I, Barabasi A-L. Human disease classification in the postgenomic era: a complex systems approach to human pathobiology. Mol Syst Biol. 2007;3:124.
3. Kitano H. Biological robustness. Nat Rev Genet. 2004;5:826–37.

Chapter 2
Theoretical Foundations of Adjustment Cord Theory

2.1 Disease as a Tension-Structured System

Biological systems are commonly described in terms of components and interactions. Genes, proteins, cells, and pathways are identified, measured, and connected through increasingly detailed models. While this component-based perspective has yielded substantial insight, it does not fully capture how complex disease systems behave under constraint.

Adjustment Cord Theory (ACT) begins from a different abstraction. Disease systems are treated as *tension-structured systems*, in which behavior emerges not from isolated elements, but from how competing demands are distributed, constrained, and resolved.

Tension, in this context, does not refer to mechanical force alone. It denotes the coexistence of incompatible requirements [1]: activation and suppression, growth and limitation, and stability and adaptability. These opposing demands are inherent to living systems and cannot be eliminated without loss of function [2].

Disease arises not when tension appears, but when its resolution becomes structurally constrained. Understanding disease therefore requires attention to how tension is allowed to move through the system and where its movement becomes restricted.

© The Author(s), under exclusive license to Springer Nature Singapore Pte Ltd. 2026

K. Komura, *Adjustment Cord Theory*,
https://doi.org/10.1007/978-981-95-7645-6_2

2.2 Horizontal Tension Lines and Convergence

In tension-structured systems, resolution does not occur vertically through hierarchical command, but horizontally through redistribution. Multiple processes operating at similar levels compete, compensate, or reinforce one another. Their interactions form *horizontal tension lines* across the system.

These lines are not pathways in the conventional sense [3]. They do not imply directional causality from upstream to downstream. Instead, they represent relational balances among processes that coexist under shared constraints.

Convergence occurs when multiple horizontal tension lines are forced to intersect at limited passages. Such convergence does not imply dominance of a single process. It reflects restriction of alternatives. The system is compelled to resolve incompatible demands through a narrow set of routes.

This notion of convergence differs from centrality [4]. A convergent passage may involve modest activity and limited connectivity, yet exert decisive influence because it constrains how tension can be resolved.

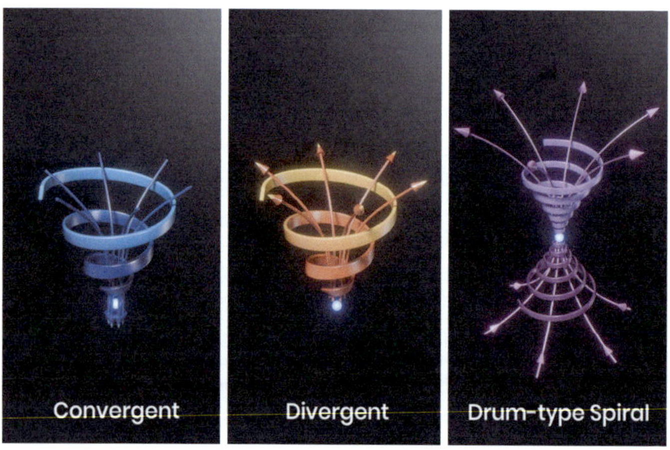

2.3 Relationship to Robustness and Systems Biology

The concept of robustness has been central to systems biology. Robust systems maintain function despite perturbation through redundancy, feedback, and adaptive reconfiguration [1]. Disease systems often exhibit remarkable robustness, preserving their behavior even under aggressive intervention.

Adjustment Cord Theory does not contradict this view. It builds upon it.

Robustness explains why systems resist change. Adjustment Cord Theory addresses where that resistance is structurally concentrated. Robustness distributes tension across alternatives. Adjustment cords emerge where those alternatives narrow.

In this sense, adjustment cords are not failures of robustness. They are its consequences. A system capable of absorbing perturbation through multiple routes will necessarily impose constraints on how those routes intersect. These constraints define passages of necessity [5]. Thus, robustness provides the background condition under which adjustment cords become meaningful.

2.4 Relationship to Network Medicine

Network medicine reframed disease as perturbations of interaction networks rather than dysfunction of isolated components [1]. This shift revealed the importance of connectivity, modules, and disease neighborhoods.

Adjustment Cord Theory aligns with this relational perspective while diverging in emphasis. Network representations describe *where interactions occur*. Adjustment cords concern *where interactions cannot be bypassed*.

High connectivity and centrality identify regions of activity and influence, but they do not guarantee necessity. A system may route tension around highly connected nodes if alternative paths remain available. Conversely, passages with modest connectivity may exert disproportionate influence if they constrain redistribution.

ACT therefore treats network analysis as a representational tool rather than a determinant of structural necessity. Networks map possibilities [6], whereas adjustment cords indicate where such possibilities become constrained into obligations.

2.5 Convergence Without Dominance

A central premise of Adjustment Cord Theory is that convergence does not imply dominance. Disease systems often converge without producing a single controlling element. Multiple processes may remain active, none exerting hierarchical control, yet the system's behavior becomes tightly constrained.

This form of convergence explains why interventions targeting dominant components frequently fail to produce durable change. Dominance reflects visibility. Necessity reflects constraint.

By distinguishing these properties, Adjustment Cord Theory provides a framework for understanding why complexity persists even when major drivers are identified and manipulated.

2.6 Positioning the Theory

Adjustment Cord Theory does not seek to replace mechanistic models, network analysis, or robustness theory. It occupies a different analytical level.

Mechanistic models explain how processes operate. Network models describe how processes are connected. Robustness theory explains why systems resist perturbation.

Adjustment Cord Theory addresses *where constraint emerges within this landscape* and how it shapes behavior, adaptation, and intervention.

By focusing on necessity rather than influence, the theory offers a complementary perspective that remains compatible with existing approaches while addressing their shared limitations.

References

1. Kitano H. Biological robustness. Nat Rev Genet. 2004;5:826–37.
2. Ingber DE. Tensegrity I. Cell structure and hierarchical systems biology. J Cell Sci. 2003;116:1157–73.
3. Barabási A-L, Oltvai ZN. Network biology: understanding the cell's functional organization. Nat Rev Genet. 2004;5:101–13.
4. Borgatti S. The network paradigm in organizational research: a review and typology. J Manag. 2003;29:991–1013.
5. Csete ME, Doyle JC. Reverse engineering of biological complexity. Science. 2002;295:1664–9.
6. Menche J, et al. Uncovering disease-disease relationships through the incomplete interactome. Science. 2015;347:1257601.

Chapter 3
Three Fundamental Morphologies of Disease Expression

3.1 Why Morphology Precedes Mechanism

Before asking how disease operates, it is necessary to ask how it appears. Disease presents itself through patterns of expression: spatial distribution, temporal behavior, and relational imbalance. These patterns are often described after mechanisms are assumed, but they can be observed independently of mechanistic explanation. Biological form often reflects optimization under constraint rather than accumulation of mechanistic detail, as exemplified by universal scaling relationships observed across biological systems [1].

Adjustment Cord Theory (ACT) begins with morphology not because form is sufficient, but because it is prior. Morphology captures how tension manifests before its routes are identified. It reflects constraint without specifying cause.

This chapter introduces three fundamental morphologies of disease expression. They are not disease categories, stages, or outcomes. They describe recurrent ways in which tension becomes visible under constraint.

At this stage, these morphologies are presented without justification.

© The Author(s), under exclusive license to Springer Nature Singapore Pte Ltd. 2026

K. Komura, *Adjustment Cord Theory*,
https://doi.org/10.1007/978-981-95-7645-6_3

3.2 Divergent Expression: Distributed Tension with Expanding Options

The first morphology is Divergent Expression. In this configuration, tension is widely distributed across the system without clear convergence. Multiple processes contribute incrementally, and no single passage appears to dominate resolution.

Divergent Expression is characterized by variability, gradual change, and broad responsiveness. Interventions often produce partial effects that dissipate across the system. Adaptation is frequent, and stability is maintained through redistribution rather than through focal control.

This morphology does not imply mild disease or low activity. Rather, it reflects a system in which alternatives remain available. Tension can move without being forced through a narrow passage.

Divergent Expression often invites mechanistic overinterpretation. Because many components appear involved, explanatory effort tends to fragment. Adjustment Cord Theory treats this morphology as structurally open rather than mechanistically complex.

3.3 Convergent Expression: Focal Resolution Under Constraint

The second morphology is convergent expression. Here, multiple tension lines are forced toward a limited set of passages. The system retains diversity of activity, yet resolution becomes focal.

Convergent expression is marked by apparent centralization. Certain regions, interfaces, or processes become repeatedly implicated, not because they dominate activity, but because alternatives have narrowed.

Intervention in convergent systems often produces disproportionate effects, both positive and negative. Small perturbations may induce significant reorganization. Conversely, strong interventions misaligned with the convergent passage may provoke compensation elsewhere.

This morphology is easily mistaken for dominance. Adjustment Cord Theory emphasizes that convergence reflects constraint, not control.

3.4 Drum-Type Expression: Convergence with Re-divergence

The third morphology is Drum-type Expression. In this configuration, tension alternates between competing passages without settling into a single resolution. The system remains bounded, yet unstable.

Drum-type Expression is characterized by fluctuation, recurrence, and apparent contradiction. Interventions may succeed temporarily, only to be followed by rebound or reversal. Competing processes alternately constrain one another, preventing collapse but also preventing resolution.

This morphology is not transitional by default. Oscillation may persist indefinitely if reciprocal constraints remain balanced. Stability is achieved through motion rather than fixation.

From an ACT perspective, Drum-type Expression reflects constrained choice rather than instability. The system is limited to a small set of alternatives and cycles among them. Oscillatory or recurrent configurations need not represent transitional instability, but may reflect stable self-organized states maintained far from equilibrium [2].

3.5 Morphologies Are Not Categories

Complex systems often exhibit a limited repertoire of emergent forms despite vast underlying diversity, suggesting that morphology reflects structural universality under constraint rather than categorical distinction [3].

The three morphologies described here do not define disease entities. A single disease may exhibit different morphologies across time, context, or scale. Morphologies may coexist, overlap, or transform into one another.

They also do not imply severity, prognosis, or therapeutic preference. Their purpose is descriptive rather than prescriptive.

Morphology precedes mechanism, but it does not replace it. These forms provide a lens through which subsequent structural analysis becomes possible. They prepare the ground for identifying where constraint emerges and where adjustment cords may reside.

The justification for these morphologies will be developed in later chapters. For now, they serve as orientation rather than explanation.

References

1. West GB, Brown JH, Enquist BJ. A general model for the origin of Allometric scaling Laws in biology. Science. 1997;276:122–6.
2. Othmer HG. Self-organization in nonequilibrium Systems (G. Nicolis and I. Prigogine). SIAM Rev. 1982;24:483–5.
3. Goldenfeld N, Kadanoff LP. Simple lessons from complexity. Science. 1999;284:87–9.

Chapter 4
From Morphology to Structure

4.1 Conceptual Transition

The three morphologies introduced in the previous chapter—*divergent, convergent, and drum-type*—are not classifications of disease entities. They are expressions of tension.

At the level of morphology, disease presents itself through visible, measurable, or intuitively recognizable patterns. These patterns often precede mechanistic understanding and, in many cases, persist even when mechanistic explanations remain incomplete or contested. Clinical intuition frequently operates at this level, recognizing stability, progression, or imminent transition before molecular evidence becomes available.

However, morphology alone does not explain why certain interventions succeed or fail. Nor does it reveal *where* within a complex system intervention should be applied. To address these questions, morphology must be translated into structure.

© The Author(s), under exclusive license to Springer Nature Singapore Pte Ltd. 2026

K. Komura, *Adjustment Cord Theory*,
https://doi.org/10.1007/978-981-95-7645-6_4

This chapter marks a conceptual shift: from how disease appears to how disease is organized.

4.2 Translating Visible Patterns into Latent Architectures

Morphological patterns emerge from underlying structures, but the relationship between the two is not one-to-one. Similar visible configurations may arise from distinct internal organizations, while markedly different clinical appearances can be generated by structurally related systems under different constraints as described in nonequilibrium and self-organizing systems [1, 2].

In Adjustment Cord Theory (ACT), structure is defined not by the presence of specific components, but by the arrangement of tensions among them. These tensions may arise from molecular interactions, cellular communication, tissue-level feedback, or environmental perturbations. What matters is not their origin, but their relational configuration.

To translate morphology into structure, three principles are essential.

First, structure is relational.

Disease states cannot be adequately described by isolated elements, even if those elements appear dominant. A molecule, cell type, or pathway acquires significance only through its position within a tension network. Structural analysis therefore shifts attention from components to relationships.

Second, structure is constrained.

Not all configurations are possible. Biological systems operate within physical, energetic, and regulatory limits. These constraints shape the pathways through which tension can propagate and converge. Adjustment cords arise precisely at points where such constraints narrow the space of possible configurations.

Third, structure is latent.

Unlike morphology, structure is not directly observable. It must be inferred from indirect evidence: network topology, temporal behavior, response to perturbation, and reproducibility across contexts. This latent nature explains why structurally critical passages are often overlooked in conventional analyses.

Through this translation, diffuse morphologies correspond to broadly distributed tension architectures without dominant constraints, convergent morphologies reflect focal restriction of tension pathways, and drum-shaped morphologies indicate balanced systems in which opposing tensions stabilize each other through resonance rather than suppression.

This mapping does not aim to replace mechanism. Instead, it provides a scaffold upon which mechanisms can be meaningfully positioned. Structure does not explain disease; it explains *where explanation becomes relevant.*

4.3 Network Representations of Disease States

Once disease structure is acknowledged as relational and latent, the challange is to approximate it without collapsing it into oversimplified components. Network representations offer a practical, though necessarily incomplete, response to this challenge.

In contemporary biomedical research, disease networks are commonly constructed from gene regulatory interactions, protein–protein associations, signaling cascades, or intercellular communication maps. These representations have contributed substantially to our understanding of disease complexity by shifting attention away from single factors toward patterns of interaction [3].

Within Adjustment Cord Theory, however, networks are not treated as explanatory endpoints. They function instead as provisional projections of an underlying tension system.

A network captures *who is connected to whom*, but not *why those connections matter at a particular moment*. The relevance of an interaction is not intrinsic to the edge itself; it emerges from how tension propagates through the network under specific constraints. Consequently, identical network topologies may correspond to fundamentally different disease states depending on temporal context, boundary conditions, and external perturbations [4].

This distinction clarifies a recurring limitation of network-based analyses. High connectivity, centrality, or statistical significance does not necessarily indicate structural leverage [5]. Many nodes appear prominent because they participate broadly, not because they constrain system behavior. In ACT terms, these nodes often function as distributors of tension, rather than as passages through which tension must pass.

To remain useful, network representations must therefore be interpreted with restraint. They are best understood as maps of potential tension pathways, not as definitive descriptions of disease organization. Their value lies in revealing relational possibilities, narrowing hypothesis space, and identifying regions where structural constraints might plausibly emerge.

Importantly, Adjustment Cord Theory does not privilege any single type of network. Gene-centric, protein-centric, and cell-centric representations each illuminate different layers of organization, yet none alone is sufficient. Structural relevance arises only when multiple representations converge on a shared passage-like configuration—one that remains stable across perturbations and contexts.

Thus, networks function as an intermediate language between morphology and structure. They translate visible patterns into analyzable forms, while still requiring theoretical guidance to distinguish structural necessity from statistical prominence.

In this sense, networks do not identify adjustment cords. They indicate where adjustment cords may exist.

4.4 Hubs, Modules, and Pseudo-centers

In network-based analyses of disease, certain elements repeatedly attract attention because of their apparent prominence. Nodes with high degree, strong centrality, or broad connectivity are often labeled as hubs and implicitly treated as key drivers of pathology. Modules with dense internal connections are similarly regarded as functional cores. While these concepts are analytically useful, their interpretation frequently exceeds what the structure itself justifies.

Adjustment Cord Theory draws a clear distinction between prominence and necessity.

A hub is prominent because it connects to many elements. A module is prominent because its components interact intensively. Neither property alone implies that the system must pass through that element in order to function or to change. Prominence describes visibility within a network representation; it does not guarantee structural leverage over system behavior. From the perspective of robustness theory, such prominence often reflects distributed buffering and adaptive redundancy rather than structural obligation [6].

This distinction becomes evident when interventions are considered. Many highly connected nodes can be perturbed with surprisingly limited system-wide impact. Such behavior is consistent with prior observations in complex engineered and biological systems, where highly connected or functionally important components often enhance robustness rather than determine points of fragility [7]. As a result, the network adapts, reroutes, or compensates. Alternative pathways absorb the perturbation, and the overall disease state remains largely unchanged. In such cases, the apparent centrality of the node reflects its distributive role rather than its constraining role.

From the perspective of Adjustment Cord Theory, truly consequential structures are not those that distribute interactions widely, but those that constrain the flow of tension. An adjustment cord is not defined by how many connections it has, but by whether tension must pass through it in order for the system to maintain its configuration. If tension can bypass a node without altering the overall state, that node is not an adjustment cord, regardless of its statistical prominence.

Modules pose a similar challenge. Dense clusters of interaction often appear to represent functional units, yet their internal cohesion does not necessarily translate into system-level control. Many modules behave as local resonators, amplifying or buffering signals without determining the global configuration. When such modules are mistaken for structural centers, they function as pseudo-centers: regions that appear central in representation but remain peripheral in terms of constraint.

Pseudo-centers arise naturally in complex systems. They are stable, reproducible, and often biologically meaningful. However, they do not define the passage points through which disease behavior is organized. Confusing pseudo-centers with adjustment cords leads to interventions that are mechanistically elegant yet structurally ineffective.

The distinction between hubs, modules, and adjustment cords therefore requires a shift in analytical focus. Rather than asking which elements are most connected or most active, the relevant question becomes which passages cannot be bypassed without reorganizing the system. This question cannot be answered by topology alone. It requires examining how the system responds to perturbation, how configurations persist over time, and how constraints limit alternative pathways.

In this framework, hubs and modules retain their descriptive value, but their role is recontextualized. They are indicators of interaction density and functional activity, not guarantors of leverage. Adjustment cords, by contrast, may appear modest, transient, or context-dependent in network representations, yet exert disproportionate influence because they define where tension is forced to converge.

Recognizing this distinction is essential for moving from descriptive complexity to actionable insight. Without it, network analysis risks mistaking visibility for control and mistaking activity for necessity.

4.5 Why Prominence Is Not Equivalent to Leverage

The analyses presented in this chapter converge on a single consequential distinction:

> What appears prominent within a system is not necessarily what exerts leverage over its behavior.

Morphology highlights visible patterns of disease expression. Network representations project relational density and interaction frequency. Hubs and modules emerge naturally from these projections, drawing attention through their scale, connectivity, or apparent activity. Each of these perspectives contributes valuable information. Yet none, on its own, identifies where meaningful intervention becomes possible.

4.5.1 Prominence Is a Property of Representation

Leverage Is a Property of Constraint

From the perspective of network theory, this distinction is not accidental. Measures such as degree, centrality, or betweenness describe positional visibility within a representation, but they do not, by themselves, confer causal or structural leverage over system behavior [5].

A prominent element is one that is frequently involved, widely connected, or statistically enriched. Such elements are easy to detect and easy to discuss. By contrast, leverage resides in locations where the system has limited alternatives. These locations may not be highly connected, highly active, or even stable across contexts. Their defining feature is not visibility, but necessity.

This distinction explains a recurring paradox in complex disease research. Targets that appear central often yield disappointing therapeutic effects, while modest or context-dependent interventions occasionally produce disproportionate change. The discrepancy does not reflect analytical failure, but conceptual misalignment. The system is being perturbed at points of visibility rather than at points of constraint. From the standpoint of biological robustness, such outcomes are not anomalous; complex systems are structured to preserve their overall behavior through redundancy and adaptive reconfiguration, even when prominent components are perturbed [6].

Adjustment Cord Theory resolves this misalignment by shifting the analytical question. Instead of asking which components dominate the system, it asks where tension is forced to pass in order for the system to maintain its configuration.

Leverage emerges not from accumulation, but from restriction. An intervention is effective not because it suppresses the largest signal, but because it alters the passage through which multiple tensions must converge.

Importantly, this reframing does not reject existing analytical tools. Morphological assessment, network analysis, and modular decomposition remain indispensable. What changes is their interpretation. Each method illuminates a different projection of the same underlying structure, yet none can, in isolation, reveal leverage. Structural necessity appears only when these projections are considered together and evaluated through their response to perturbation and persistence over time.

From this perspective, adjustment cords are neither dominant controllers nor universal regulators. They are structurally imposed passages that emerge from the constraints of the system itself. Their influence is conditional, context-sensitive, and often invisible to static analysis. Precisely because of these properties, they are frequently overlooked.

Recognizing that prominence is not equivalent to leverage marks a decisive step in moving from descriptive complexity to actionable understanding. It clarifies why certain interventions fail despite strong rationale, why others succeed unexpectedly, and why effective intervention requires attention not only to what is present, but to what cannot be bypassed.

With this distinction established, the subsequent chapters will move beyond structural description toward dynamics and intervention. The focus will shift from identifying components to understanding how configurations change and how adjustment cords can be engaged without destabilizing the system they constrain.

References

1. Othmer HG. Self-organization in nonequilibrium systems (G. Nicolis and I. Prigogine). SIAM Rev. 1982;24:483–5.
2. Goldenfeld N, Kadanoff LP. Simple lessons from complexity. Science. 1999;284:87–9.
3. Barabási A-L, Oltvai ZN. Network biology: understanding the cell's functional organization. Nat Rev Genet. 2004;5:101–13.
4. Menche J, et al. Uncovering disease-disease relationships through the incomplete interactome. Science. 2015;347:1257601.
5. Borgatti S. The network paradigm in organizational research: a review and typology. J Manag. 2003;29:991–1013.
6. Kitano H. Biological robustness. Nat Rev Genet. 2004;5:826–37.
7. Csete ME, Doyle JC. Reverse engineering of biological complexity. Science. 2002;295:1664–9.

Chapter 5
Defining the Adjustment Cord

5.1 Why a Precise Definition Is Necessary

Up to this point, adjustment cords have been described implicitly—as passages through which tension must pass when alternatives narrow. This description is intentionally provisional. Without a precise definition, however, the concept risks being absorbed into existing categories such as hubs, drivers, bottlenecks, or biomarkers.

This risk is not trivial. In complex systems research, new terms are often introduced to rename familiar structures rather than to distinguish fundamentally different ones. When this occurs, conceptual novelty is mistaken for explanatory progress, and analytical clarity is lost.

Adjustment Cord Theory does not introduce a new label for importance. It introduces a criterion for necessity.

A precise definition is therefore required not to expand the concept, but to constrain it. Only by specifying what qualifies—and what does not—can adjustment cords function as anchors for analysis rather than as flexible metaphors. Without such boundaries, any prominent, influential, or therapeutically relevant element could be retroactively designated as an adjustment cord, rendering the concept vacuous.

© The Author(s), under exclusive license to Springer Nature Singapore Pte Ltd. 2026

K. Komura, *Adjustment Cord Theory*,
https://doi.org/10.1007/978-981-95-7645-6_5

Moreover, necessity cannot be inferred from appearance alone. Visibility, activity, connectivity, and statistical association are properties of representation. Structural necessity is a property of constraint. Confusing the two leads to interventions that are well justified within their own analytical frames yet fail to alter system behavior in durable ways.

This chapter therefore establishes a formal definition of the adjustment cord and delineates its boundary conditions. The aim is not to close interpretation, but to prevent misalignment. By clarifying what an adjustment cord is—and what it is not—the theory preserves its capacity to distinguish leverage from prominence and obligation from influence.

The sections that follow proceed accordingly: first by defining the adjustment cord conceptually, then by contrasting it with related constructs, and finally by addressing patterns of false convergence that obscure structural necessity.

5.2 Conceptual Definition and Boundary Conditions

An adjustment cord is defined as a structurally imposed passage within a complex system through which tension must pass in order for the system to maintain or transition its configuration.

This definition has several implications.

First, an adjustment cord is not defined by its components. It may involve a molecule, a cell population, an interaction interface, or a regulatory process. None of these elements qualifies as an adjustment cord by identity alone. What matters is whether the system is forced to route tension through that passage under the constraints of the system.

Second, an adjustment cord is not defined by activity or magnitude. High expression, strong signaling, or statistical enrichment does not establish an adjustment cord. A passage may exert decisive influence despite low baseline activity, while highly active elements may be bypassed without altering the system state.

Third, an adjustment cord is context-dependent but not arbitrary. Its relevance emerges under specific configurations of constraint, yet it is not freely chosen by the observer. If a passage repeatedly appears as unavoidable across perturbations, temporal shifts, or representational layers, it reflects structural necessity rather than analytical coincidence. Boundary conditions are therefore essential to prevent conceptual drift. A structure qualifies as an adjustment cord only if the following conditions are met.

The system cannot preserve its configuration if the passage is disrupted. Alternative pathways exist but are insufficient to compensate without reorganization. The passage remains relevant across observational modalities or perturbative contexts.

If any of these conditions fail, the structure may still be biologically meaningful, but it does not function as an adjustment cord.

This definition deliberately excludes many entities commonly targeted in disease research. Drivers that can be bypassed, hubs that distribute without constraining, and biomarkers that reflect but do not shape system behavior all fall outside the scope of adjustment cords.

By enforcing these boundaries, Adjustment Cord Theory resists conceptual inflation. The adjustment cord is not a metaphor for importance. It is a designation for necessity imposed by structure. An adjustment cord should not be conflated with a node in a network representation. A node is a representational unit defined by identity or connectivity, an adjustment cord is a structurally imposed passage defined by necessity. A cord may intersect one or more nodes, but it is not reducible to any single node.

5.3 Adjustment Cords Versus Drivers, Hubs, and Biomarkers

To function as an analytical tool rather than a rhetorical device, the concept of the adjustment cord must be distinguished explicitly from entities that are already well established in disease research. Without such distinction, adjustment cords risk being conflated with drivers, hubs, bottlenecks, or biomarkers, thereby losing their conceptual specificity.

Drivers are elements whose perturbation alters disease behavior under certain conditions. They often occupy upstream positions in signaling hierarchies or exert strong regulatory influence. While drivers can be therapeutically relevant, their influence is conditional. Many drivers can be bypassed through alternative pathways or compensated for by system-level adaptation. Such bypass and compensation are well-recognized features of biologically robust systems, in which function is preserved through redundancy and adaptive reconfiguration rather than reliance on single dominant drivers [1]. A driver that can be circumvented without reorganizing the system does not constitute an adjustment cord.

Hubs are defined by connectivity. Their prominence arises from the number or strength of their interactions rather than from structural necessity. Hubs frequently serve as distributors, spreading signals or resources across the system. This role confers visibility but not inevitability. If tension can be rerouted around a hub while preserving the overall configuration, the hub does not function as an adjustment cord, regardless of its centrality metrics. This limitation of connectivity-based importance has been emphasized in network theory, where centrality measures capture positional visibility rather than structural inevitability [2]. Biomarkers occupy a different category altogether. They reflect system states rather than constrain them. A biomarker may correlate strongly with disease activity, prognosis, or treatment response, yet exert no influence on the organization of the system itself. Such markers are valuable for observation and stratification, but they do not define passages through which tension must pass.

These distinctions underscore a critical point. Adjustment cords are not identified by what happens when they are perturbed, but by what happens when the system attempts to function without them. If the system cannot maintain or transition its configuration without reorganizing around a given passage, that passage meets the criterion of structural necessity.

This criterion also clarifies why adjustment cords are often overlooked. They may not sit upstream, may not appear highly connected, and may not produce strong signals under baseline conditions. Their relevance becomes apparent only when constraints tighten and alternatives disappear. Under such conditions, the system reveals which passages it cannot avoid.

Importantly, an adjustment cord is not superior to drivers, hubs, or biomarkers. It serves a different analytical purpose. Drivers explain influence, hubs explain connectivity, and biomarkers explain correlation. Adjustment cords explain necessity. Confusing these categories leads to interventions that are well motivated yet structurally misaligned.

By maintaining this separation, Adjustment Cord Theory preserves conceptual clarity. The adjustment cord is not a general term for importance. It is a precise designation for passages imposed by structure, revealed by constraint, and confirmed by the system's inability to bypass them.

5.4 False Convergence and Misleading Intervention Points

In complex disease systems, intervention strategies often converge repeatedly on the same types of targets. These targets are selected not because they are structurally unavoidable, but because multiple analytical perspectives appear to point toward them simultaneously. This phenomenon can be described as false convergence.

False convergence occurs when distinct observational layers align superficially without reflecting structural necessity.

A molecule may appear highly expressed, centrally connected in a network, and strongly associated with clinical outcomes. Each observation is valid within its own framework. The error arises when their coincidence is interpreted as evidence of an unavoidable passage.

Such convergence is persuasive because it feels confirmatory. Independent analyses seem to reinforce one another, creating the impression that the system has revealed its core. In reality, these analyses may be capturing the same distributive feature from different angles rather than identifying a constraining structure. Similar forms of apparent convergence have been described in analyses of complex engineered and biological systems, where agreement across methods reflects shared assumptions rather than true points of structural fragility [3].

Adjustment Cord Theory treats this pattern with caution. Convergence of signals does not imply convergence of constraint. A system can amplify activity around a region precisely because that region is flexible, redundant, or capable of absorbing perturbation. In such cases, prominence reflects adaptability rather than necessity.

Misleading intervention points often emerge from this misinterpretation. Targets selected under false convergence may respond predictably to perturbation yet fail to induce durable system-level change. The system adjusts locally while preserving its global configuration. Repeated cycles of apparent success followed by relapse or compensation are characteristic outcomes.

False convergence is further reinforced by methodological coupling. Many analytical tools share underlying assumptions, data sources, or preprocessing steps. As a result, agreement across methods may reflect shared bias rather than independent confirmation. Such coupling effects have been widely discussed in the context of methodological bias and nonindependence across analytical pipelines [4]. Without an explicit criterion for necessity, such agreement is easily mistaken for structural insight.

Adjustment cords, by contrast, are revealed not by agreement at baseline, but by persistence under constraint. When alternative pathways narrow, when compensatory mechanisms fail, and when the system is forced to reorganize, the passages that remain unavoidable become visible. These passages may not have been prominent under unconstrained conditions.

Recognizing false convergence requires a shift in evaluative logic. The relevant question is no longer whether multiple analyses highlight the same element, but whether the system can function without reorganizing around that element. Only the latter allows structural necessity from analytical coincidence.

By making this distinction explicit, Adjustment Cord Theory provides a framework for interpreting convergence without being misled by it. Convergence is not dismissed, but reclassified. It is treated as a signal that warrants further structural testing, not as a conclusion in itself.

5.5 Adjustment Cords as Necessary but Nondominant Structures

A defining characteristic of adjustment cords is that they exert necessity without dominance. This property distinguishes them not only from drivers and hubs but also from many structures that are traditionally considered central to disease behavior.

Dominant structures attract attention by their scale, activity, or persistence. They shape observable dynamics and often define the language through which disease is discussed.

Adjustment cords, by contrast, do not dominate system behavior in an overt manner. They do not amplify signals, enforce directionality, or impose control across the system. Their influence is quieter and more restrictive.

This distinction is essential. Dominance operates through magnitude, while necessity operates through limitation. This distinction is consistent with robustness theory, which emphasizes that system behavior is preserved not by dominant components but by constraint-aware organization, redundancy, and adaptive reconfiguration [1]. An adjustment cord constrains what the system can do, not by overwhelming it, but by restricting the available paths through which tension can be resolved. The system may appear flexible and adaptive until it encounters such a constraint. At that point, the importance of the passage becomes apparent.

Because of this property, adjustment cords are often invisible to analyses focused on steady-state behavior. Under unconstrained conditions, the system distributes tension across multiple pathways, masking the role of any single passage. Only when constraints intensify—through progression, perturbation, or intervention—does the system reveal which passages it cannot bypass. Analyses of complex engineered and biological systems have similarly shown that structurally critical elements often reveal their importance only under constraint, remaining inconspicuous under unconstrained or steady-state conditions [3].

This behavior explains why adjustment cords may appear transient, context-dependent, or weakly expressed. Their relevance is not constant, but conditional. Yet this conditionality does not imply fragility. On the contrary, it reflects structural embedding. A passage that becomes unavoidable only under constraint is more deeply integrated into system organization than one that is merely active at baseline.

Recognizing adjustment cords therefore requires tolerance for subtlety. The absence of dominance should not be mistaken for irrelevance. Nor should variability across contexts be interpreted as inconsistency. Adjustment cords are stable in function, not in appearance. Their role is defined by what the system cannot do without them, rather than by what they continuously impose.

This perspective also reframes therapeutic ambition. Effective intervention does not require suppressing the most active element or dismantling the most visible structure. It requires engaging the passage that the system relies on when its options narrow. Such engagement may not produce immediate or dramatic effects, but it alters the conditions under which the system can maintain its configuration.

In this sense, adjustment cords are points of obligation rather than control. They do not command the system; they delimit it. Their significance lies not in how much they act, but in how little the system can act without them.

With this distinction established, the focus can now shift from definition to dynamics. The following chapter will examine how adjustment cords emerge, disappear, or relocate as system configurations change over time and how intervention reshapes the landscape of constraint itself.

5.6 Implications of Structural Necessity

Defining adjustment cords as necessary but nondominant structures has implications that extend beyond classification. It reshapes how causality, intervention, and failure are interpreted in complex disease systems.

First, structural necessity reframes causation. In systems governed by constraint, causality is not localized to a single component or event. Instead, it is distributed across configurations that limit how tension can be resolved. Adjustment cords do not cause disease states in isolation; they delimit the configurations through which disease states persist or change.

Causation, in this sense, is enacted through restriction rather than initiation.

Second, this perspective alters how intervention is evaluated. Traditional approaches often assess efficacy by the magnitude or immediacy of response. Structural interventions may not satisfy these expectations. Engaging an adjustment cord can produce delayed, indirect, or modest effects, yet fundamentally alter the system's future trajectories. The absence of dramatic short-term change does not imply ineffectiveness; it may indicate that the system is being reconfigured rather than overridden.

Third, structural necessity clarifies the meaning of failure. When interventions targeting prominent elements fail to produce durable change, the outcome is frequently attributed to resistance, redundancy, or complexity beyond control. From the perspective of Adjustment Cord Theory, such failures often reflect misalignment between the site of intervention and the location of constraint. The system does not resist intervention; it accommodates it.

Finally, recognizing structural necessity imposes methodological discipline. Claims of leverage must be supported not by prominence or correlation, but by evidence that a passage cannot be bypassed without reorganization. This requirement shifts emphasis from static association to dynamic testing—probing how systems respond as options narrow, compensatory mechanisms falter, and configurations are forced to change.

Together, these implications prepare the ground for the next phase of analysis. Having established what adjustment cords are, what they are not, and why they matter, the focus can now move from definition to dynamics. The following chapter examines how adjustment cords emerge, migrate, or dissolve over time and how intervention reshapes the landscape of constraint within which disease unfolds.

References

1. Kitano H. Biological robustness. Nat Rev Genet. 2004;5:826–37.
2. Borgatti S. The network paradigm in organizational research: a review and typology. J Manag. 2003;29:991–1013.
3. Csete ME, Doyle JC. Reverse engineering of biological complexity. Science. 2002;295:1664–9.
4. Ioannidis JPA. Why Most published research findings are false. PLoS Med. 2005;2:e124.

Chapter 6
Dynamic Reconfiguration of Tension Networks

6.1 From Structure to Dynamics

The definition of an adjustment cord establishes what is structurally necessary within a given configuration. Yet disease systems are not static. They evolve, adapt, and reorganize over time in response to internal progression and external perturbation. As a result, the location and relevance of adjustment cords cannot be assumed to be fixed.

This chapter shifts the analytical focus from structure as a snapshot to structure as a trajectory. The central question is no longer where tension must pass at a given moment, but how the pathways of tension are reshaped as system configurations change.

Dynamic reconfiguration does not imply instability in a general sense. Many disease states persist precisely because their underlying constraints are robust. However, robustness does not preclude change. It determines the manner in which change becomes possible.

Adjustment Cord Theory (ACT) approaches dynamics not as continuous fluctuation, but as reorganization under constraint. What changes is not the presence of tension, but the routes through which it is allowed to pass.

© The Author(s), under exclusive license to Springer Nature Singapore Pte Ltd. 2026

K. Komura, *Adjustment Cord Theory*,
https://doi.org/10.1007/978-981-95-7645-6_6

6.2 Temporal Instability and Phase Transitions

Disease progression is often described in terms of accumulation or escalation. From the perspective of tension networks, however, progression is better understood as a sequence of constrained reconfigurations. The system does not simply intensify its existing behavior; it reorganizes the pathways through which tension is distributed.

Temporal instability arises when previously available pathways lose their capacity to absorb or redistribute tension. This loss may result from gradual change, such as chronic stress on regulatory mechanisms, or from discrete events, such as therapeutic intervention or environmental perturbation. When such changes occur, the system is forced to reroute tension through alternative passages.

Phase transitions mark moments when this rerouting can no longer preserve the existing configuration. At these points, the system reorganizes its structure, often abruptly. The clinical manifestation of such transitions may appear sudden, yet the underlying process reflects a gradual narrowing of alternatives followed by enforced reconfiguration.

Within this framework, adjustment cords are not permanent fixtures. A passage that functions as an adjustment cord in one phase may lose that role if constraints are relaxed or redistributed. Conversely, previously peripheral passages may become unavoidable as options narrow. What remains constant is not the location of the cord, but the principle that tension must pass through a limited set of routes imposed by structure.

This perspective clarifies why early and late disease states can respond differently to the same intervention. An intervention that engages an adjustment cord in one phase may bypass it entirely in another. The apparent inconsistency reflects not therapeutic failure, but structural relocation of necessity.

Temporal analysis therefore requires attention not only to what changes, but to what ceases to be possible. Phase transitions are defined less by the emergence of new activity than by the disappearance of viable alternatives. Adjustment cords become visible precisely at these moments, when the system reveals which passages it can no longer avoid.

6.3 Subtype Shifts Without Categorical Redefinition

Disease subtypes are commonly defined by observable features: clinical presentation, dominant pathways, or response patterns. These classifications are useful for communication and decision-making, yet they often obscure a critical phenomenon. Systems can undergo substantial internal reconfiguration without crossing categorical boundaries. This limitation of categorical disease classification has been noted in postgenomic and systems-based frameworks, which emphasize that shared labels may conceal substantial internal heterogeneity and reconfiguration [1].

From the perspective of Adjustment Cord Theory, subtype shifts do not require redefinition of disease identity. What changes is not the label, but the distribution of constraints within the system.

Within a given subtype, multiple configurations may be possible. These configurations share external characteristics while differing in how tension is routed internally. As long as the system can maintain its outward behavior, such internal shifts remain invisible to classification schemes. The disease appears stable, even as its structural organization evolves.

This phenomenon explains why patients with the same diagnosis and subtype may respond divergently to identical interventions. Such divergent responses within the same diagnostic category are consistent with the concept of biological robustness, whereby systems preserve outward behavior through internal reconfiguration under constraint [2]. The intervention engages different passages in different configurations, despite superficial similarity. Apparent unpredictability arises not from randomness, but from unrecognized structural diversity within categories.

Subtype shifts often occur gradually. As constraints accumulate or redistribute, certain passages become less available while others gain relevance. The system adapts by rerouting tension, preserving its categorical appearance. Only when available routes narrow beyond a threshold does overt transition occur, prompting reclassification or recognition of progression.

Adjustment cords play a central role in this process. A passage that functions as an adjustment cord in one internal configuration may be peripheral in another, even within the same subtype. Conversely, a passage that appears insignificant under baseline conditions may become unavoidable as internal alternatives diminish.

This view reframes subtype stability. Stability does not imply structural uniformity. It reflects the system's capacity to absorb change without altering its outward classification. Subtype shifts are therefore not anomalies, but expected outcomes of constrained adaptability.

Recognizing these shifts requires attention to internal reorganization rather than external markers alone. Without such attention, interventions may be timed or selected based on outdated assumptions about structural necessity. What was once an effective engagement of an adjustment cord may no longer be relevant, despite unchanged diagnostic labels.

By distinguishing categorical identity from structural configuration, Adjustment Cord Theory provides a framework for understanding variability within apparent sameness. Subtypes remain useful descriptors, but they no longer imply fixed internal organization. The decisive factor is not what the disease is called, but how its constraints are currently arranged.

6.4 External Perturbation and Internal Rearrangement

External perturbations are often introduced with the intention of correcting a specific abnormality. Therapeutic agents, environmental changes, and behavioral interventions are typically designed to suppress, enhance, or replace a particular function. From the perspective of Adjustment Cord Theory, however, the primary effect of perturbation is not correction but rearrangement. From a systems perspective, this behavior is consistent with prior observations that biological and engineered systems respond to perturbation primarily through redistribution and reconfiguration rather than linear correction [2, 3].

When a system is perturbed, tension does not disappear. It is redistributed. Pathways that were previously available may be weakened or blocked, while alternative routes become more heavily utilized. This redistribution can stabilize the system, destabilize it, or shift it into a different configuration altogether.

Crucially, perturbations do not act on isolated elements. They act on constraints. By altering the availability of certain passages, an intervention reshapes the space of possible configurations. The system responds not by returning to a prior state, but by reorganizing itself within the new set of limitations imposed.

This perspective explains why interventions with similar intended targets can produce divergent outcomes. Such divergence is expected in robust, nonequilibrium systems, where identical perturbations may be absorbed, redirected, or amplified depending on the availability of alternative pathways and the current configuration of constraints [2]. The effect of a perturbation depends not only on what it acts upon, but on what alternatives remain accessible. An intervention that engages an adjustment cord in one configuration may simply divert tension elsewhere in another, producing compensation rather than change.

Internal rearrangement often occurs silently. Clinical markers may improve, stabilize, or fluctuate without clear indication that the underlying structure has shifted. Over time, however, these rearrangements accumulate. Pathways that repeatedly absorb redistributed tension may become reinforced, while others atrophy. The system adapts to the perturbation, not by resolving tension, but by learning new routes around it.

This adaptive response is frequently mistaken for resistance or failure. From an ACT perspective, it reflects the system's capacity to preserve its configuration under altered constraints. The intervention has not been ignored; it has been incorporated.

Importantly, external perturbation can also create new adjustment cords. By altering structural constraints, perturbations may reorganize the system in a manner analogous to architectural rebalancing in tensegrity-based structures, where local changes redistribute global stress and redefine points of necessity [4]. By closing off previously flexible routes, an intervention may force tension through passages that were once peripheral. These newly imposed necessities can become dominant determinants of subsequent behavior, including treatment response and adverse effects.

Such dynamics underscore a key implication. Interventions are not neutral probes of system behavior. They are structural events. From this standpoint, intervention resembles a structural perturbation rather than an external probe, reshaping the constraints under which adaptation occurs rather than merely revealing preexisting mechanisms [2]. Each perturbation leaves an imprint on the organization of constraints, shaping not only immediate outcomes but future possibilities.

Understanding this process requires shifting attention from short-term effects to configurational consequences. The question is not whether an intervention changes a measurable parameter, but how it alters the routes through which the system can adapt. Only by addressing this question can interventions be designed to engage necessity rather than provoke rearrangement.

6.5 When Intervention Reshapes the System Itself

Intervention is often conceived as an external force applied to an otherwise stable system. From this viewpoint, the system responds, improves, or deteriorates, while its underlying identity remains intact. Adjustment Cord Theory challenges this assumption. Certain interventions do not merely act upon the system; they become part of its structure. From the standpoint of biological robustness, persistent perturbations can be accommodated through structural reconfiguration, such that the system incorporates the intervention into its adaptive architecture rather than returning to its original state [2].

When an intervention persistently alters the availability of tension pathways, the system adapts by reorganizing its constraints. Over time, this reorganization may stabilize into a new configuration that depends on the presence of the intervention itself. At this point, the intervention no longer functions as an external perturbation. It has been incorporated into the system's architecture.

Such incorporation has several consequences. First, withdrawal of the intervention may precipitate disproportionate instability. This form of dependency is consistent with observations in complex engineered and biological systems, where adaptive compensation can stabilize new operating regimes that become fragile upon removal of the compensating constraint [3]. The system has learned to route tension through passages that exist only under the imposed constraints. Removing those constraints abruptly exposes the absence of viable alternatives.

Second, the system's future responses become conditioned by the structural changes induced by the intervention. Subsequent perturbations interact not with the original configuration, but with a reorganized one. Apparent loss of efficacy, unexpected adverse effects, or qualitative shifts in disease behavior can often be traced to this altered baseline. This process also explains paradoxical responses. Within robust systems, such paradoxical effects are not contradictory but expected, arising when suppression of a prominent pathway forces redistribution through alternative routes that were previously secondary or latent [2]. When an intervention suppresses a prominent pathway, it may force tension through less visible passages that were previously irrelevant. These passages, once activated, can dominate subsequent behavior. The resulting phenotype appears contradictory only if the intervention is viewed in isolation rather than as a structural event.

From the perspective of Adjustment Cord Theory, such outcomes are not anomalies. They are expected whenever an intervention engages constraint without accounting for the system's capacity to reorganize. The system does not resist change; it adapts to it. What appears paradoxical is the consequence of engaging the wrong level of structure.

Crucially, this does not imply that intervention should be avoided or minimized. It implies that intervention should be designed with awareness of its structural footprint. The goal is not to suppress activity indiscriminately, but to engage passages that redistribute tension without creating new, more restrictive dependencies.

This consideration reframes therapeutic success. Short-term improvement does not guarantee structural alignment, and long-term stability does not necessarily reflect resolution. Accordingly, short-term stabilization should not be conflated with structural resolution, as robust systems may preserve their overall behavior while reorganizing internally under sustained perturbation [2]. An intervention may achieve both only if it engages an adjustment cord in a manner that relaxes constraint rather than relocating it.

With this understanding, intervention is no longer a terminal act but a formative one. This formative role of intervention can be understood by analogy to tensegrity-based structures, in which local alterations redistribute global stress and redefine structural dependencies rather than producing isolated effects [4]. Each engagement reshapes the landscape of necessity, influencing which passages will matter next.

Recognizing this continuity is essential for designing strategies that alter disease trajectories rather than merely managing their manifestations.

References

1. Loscalzo J, Kohane I, Barabasi A-L. Human disease classification in the postgenomic era: a complex systems approach to human pathobiology. Mol Syst Biol. 2007;3:124.
2. Kitano H. Biological robustness. Nat Rev Genet. 2004;5:826–37.
3. Csete ME, Doyle JC. Reverse engineering of biological complexity. Science. 2002;295:1664–9.
4. Ingber DE. Tensegrity I. cell structure and hierarchical systems biology. J Cell Sci. 2003;116:1157–73.

Chapter 7
Intervention Through Adjustment Cords

7.1 From Targeting to Designing

Conventional therapeutic strategies are largely built around targeting. A component is identified, its activity is modified, and the resulting effect is evaluated. This approach presumes that influence scales with magnitude: stronger targets produce stronger outcomes.

Adjustment Cord Theory (ACT) proposes a different premise. Effective intervention does not arise from targeting the most influential component, but from engaging the structure that constrains influence itself. The task is therefore not to select a target, but to design an intervention that interacts appropriately with structural necessity.

This shift reframes intervention as a design problem rather than a selection problem. The central question becomes how to engage an adjustment cord without provoking compensatory rearrangement or creating new dependencies. Answering this question requires abandoning the assumption that more force produces better results.

© The Author(s), under exclusive license to Springer Nature Singapore Pte Ltd. 2026

K. Komura, *Adjustment Cord Theory*,
https://doi.org/10.1007/978-981-95-7645-6_7

7.2 Why Targeting Dominant Components Often Fails

Dominant components attract intervention because their effects are visible and measurable. High activity, strong associations, and reproducible signals provide a compelling rationale for action. Yet such dominance often reflects distribution rather than constraint [1, 2].

When a dominant component is perturbed, the system frequently responds by rerouting tension through alternative pathways. These alternatives may be less efficient or less visible, but they suffice to preserve the overall configuration [1, 3]. The intervention succeeds locally while failing structurally.

This pattern explains a common therapeutic trajectory. Initial response is followed by stabilization, compensation, or relapse. Each phase reflects not resistance, but adaptation. The system incorporates the intervention by reorganizing around it, leaving the underlying constraints intact.

From the perspective of Adjustment Cord Theory, this outcome is expected whenever intervention engages prominence rather than necessity. Dominant components can absorb perturbation precisely because they are embedded in flexible regions of the network. Their removal or suppression does not force reorganization at the level that determines system behavior.

This insight does not negate the value of dominant targets. Such targets may be necessary for symptom control or short--term stabilization. However, their perturbation alone is insufficient to alter disease trajectories if adjustment cords remain unengaged.

Recognizing this limitation clarifies why escalating intensity often yields diminishing returns. Increasing dose, potency, or breadth amplifies local effects without addressing the structural passage that governs adaptation [1]. The system responds proportionally, preserving its configuration while absorbing the added force.

Effective intervention therefore requires a different orientation. Rather than asking which component exerts the greatest influence, the relevant question is which passage the system cannot bypass when its options narrow. Only engagement at this level compels reorganization rather than redistribution.

7.3 Vector Mismatch and Paradoxical Effects

Interventions are not defined solely by what they target, but by the direction in which they act. Every perturbation imposes a vector upon the system: it pushes, suppresses, diverts, or amplifies tension along a particular orientation. Whether an intervention succeeds or fails depends not only on its intensity but also on how this vector aligns with the structure of constraint [1, 3].

Vector mismatch arises when the direction of intervention conflicts with the orientation of an adjustment cord. In such cases, the system does not resolve tension through the intended passage. Instead, it is forced to redirect tension into alternative routes that were previously secondary or inactive [1].

This redirection can produce effects that appear paradoxical. An intervention designed to suppress activity may provoke emergence elsewhere. A measure intended to stabilize the system may increase volatility. These outcomes are often interpreted as idiosyncratic responses or off-target effects. From the perspective of Adjustment Cord Theory, they reflect misalignment between intervention vector and structural necessity. Similar behaviors have been described in robust biological and engineered systems, where perturbations aligned against system constraints induce compensatory reorganization rather than resolution [1, 3].

Paradoxical effects are therefore not contradictions of mechanism. They are confirmations of structure. The system is responding coherently to imposed constraints by preserving its capacity to route tension, even if doing so generates unexpected manifestations [1].

Vector mismatch is most likely to occur when intervention is guided by prominence rather than necessity. Highly visible components suggest obvious directions for action, yet these directions may be orthogonal to the actual passage through which tension must flow. Suppressing such components alters surface dynamics without engaging the constraining route, forcing the system to compensate elsewhere [3].

Importantly, paradoxical effects do not require excessive force. Even modest perturbations can induce disproportionate reconfiguration if their direction conflicts with constraint. Conversely, stronger interventions aligned with an adjustment cord may produce subtle but durable change, precisely because they do not provoke compensatory diversion. Such nonlinear responses are characteristic of systems maintained far from equilibrium [4].

This distinction reframes how unintended outcomes should be interpreted. Rather than signaling failure or unpredictability, paradoxical effects indicate that the intervention has intersected the system at the wrong angle. The system is not resisting the intervention; it is adapting to it according to its structure.

Recognizing vector mismatch has practical implications. It suggests that successful intervention requires attention to orientation as much as to target selection. The question is not merely whether an element is involved, but whether acting upon it directs tension toward or away from the unavoidable passage.

Within this framework, paradoxical effects become diagnostic. They reveal the presence and orientation of constraints that were previously unrecognized. Properly interpreted, such effects can inform subsequent design by indicating where adjustment cords are not located and by narrowing the space of viable intervention vectors.

7.4 Successful Intervention as Tension Redistribution

Within Adjustment Cord Theory, successful intervention is not defined by suppression, elimination, or normalization of individual components. It is defined by how tension is redistributed within the system.

In many therapeutic frameworks, success is equated with reduction: lowering activity, decreasing burden, or removing a pathological element. While such outcomes may be desirable, they do not by themselves indicate structural alignment. A system can exhibit marked local improvement while preserving the same global constraints that generated disease behavior in the first place.

From an ACT perspective, tension cannot be destroyed. It can only be redirected, redistributed, or reorganized. The decisive question is therefore not whether tension is reduced at a given site, but whether its redistribution alters the set of unavoidable passages that govern system behavior.

A successful intervention engages an adjustment cord in a manner that relaxes constraint rather than relocating it. This relaxation may take several forms. Tension that was previously forced through a narrow passage may be dispersed across multiple routes. Alternatively, competing constraints may be rebalanced such that no single passage remains obligatory. In either case, the system gains degrees of freedom.

Such changes are often subtle. They may not produce dramatic short-term effects, and they may not correspond neatly to conventional outcome measures. Yet they manifest as increased stability, reduced sensitivity to perturbation, or diminished tendency toward abrupt transition. These features reflect structural change rather than symptomatic control.

This distinction clarifies why some interventions that appear modest can have durable impact, while others with strong immediate effects fail to alter long-term trajectories. The former modify how tension is distributed; the latter merely displace where it is expressed. Only the former reduce structural obligation.

Importantly, redistribution does not imply uniformity. Successful intervention does not aim to flatten the system or erase heterogeneity. Heterogeneity is intrinsic to complex systems. The goal is not to eliminate variation, but to prevent it from being forced through a single constraining passage.

This perspective also reframes adverse effects. An intervention that redistributes tension effectively may initially expose vulnerabilities elsewhere, producing transient instability. Such effects should not be mistaken for failure if they accompany a net relaxation of constraint. Conversely, smooth short-term responses may conceal deeper structural relocation that preserves or even intensifies obligation.

Evaluating success therefore requires attention to pattern rather than magnitude. Indicators include delayed progression, altered response to subsequent perturbation, and reduced dependence on continued intervention. These features suggest that the system is no longer organized around the same unavoidable passage.

In this sense, successful intervention is not an endpoint but a reconfiguration. It does not resolve tension; it changes how the system must live with it.

7.5 Designing Interventions for Structural Leverage

Designing intervention within Adjustment Cord Theory does not mean specifying where to act or how strongly to act. It means determining how an action interacts with structural necessity. Structural leverage arises not from force, but from alignment with constraint [3].

Three principles follow directly from this perspective.

First, leverage precedes magnitude.

An intervention that aligns with an adjustment cord may require minimal intensity to induce durable change.

Conversely, interventions applied at misaligned locations often demand escalating force without achieving reconfiguration [3]. Design therefore begins by identifying where necessity resides, not by optimizing strength.

Second, orientation matters more than specificity.

Highly specific interventions are often favored for their precision, yet specificity alone does not guarantee alignment. What matters is whether the direction imposed by the intervention engages or bypasses the constraining passage. Broad or indirect actions may exert greater leverage if they intersect the system along the correct orientation.

Third, timing is inseparable from structure.

Adjustment cords are configuration-dependent. An intervention aligned with structural necessity in one phase may be irrelevant in another. Effective design therefore requires sensitivity to when constraints tighten or relax. Timing is not an external consideration; it is part of the structural context.

These principles imply a departure from intervention as isolated decision-making. Each action reshapes the landscape of constraint and thereby alters what will be necessary next. Design must therefore account for sequences, not single moves. Structural leverage is achieved by anticipating how the system will reorganize in response to engagement.

This approach also clarifies why uniform strategies fail across heterogeneous systems. Structural leverage is not universal; it is contextual [3]. The same intervention may engage necessity in one configuration and miss it entirely in another. Designing for leverage thus requires continuous reassessment of constraint rather than adherence to fixed targets.

Importantly, designing for structural leverage does not imply full control. Complex systems cannot be commanded. They can only be guided by altering the conditions under which adaptation occurs. The aim is not to dictate outcomes, but to expand the space of viable configurations.

In this sense, intervention becomes an act of structural negotiation. By engaging adjustment cords thoughtfully, it is possible to relax obligation without provoking compensatory restriction elsewhere. Such negotiation favors durability over immediacy and coherence over force.

With these principles in place, the discussion can move beyond individual interventions toward broader generalization. The next chapter will examine how these design concepts apply across disease classes without collapsing into disease-specific prescriptions.

References

1. Kitano H. Biological robustness. Nat Rev Genet. 2004;5:826–37.
2. Borgatti S. The network paradigm in organizational research: a review and typology. J Manag. 2003;29:991–1013.
3. Csete ME, Doyle JC. Reverse engineering of biological complexity. Science. 2002;295:1664–9.
4. Othmer HG. Self-organization in nonequilibrium systems (G. Nicolis and I. Prigogine). SIAM Rev. 1982;24:483–5.

Chapter 8
Structural Motifs, Generality, and Transferability

8.1 Why Disease-Specific Detail Is Deliberately Minimized

Adjustment Cord Theory is not intended to function as a comprehensive explanatory framework for individual diseases. Its purpose is to clarify how constraint, necessity, and redistribution recur across heterogeneous systems. For this reason, disease-specific detail is deliberately minimized at this stage of exposition.

Detailed pathological descriptions, molecular mechanisms, and therapeutic protocols are indispensable for clinical practice and disease-focused research. However, when introduced prematurely, such detail can obscure structural regularities by anchoring interpretation to familiar categories. The present chapter therefore suspends disease specificity in order to preserve conceptual clarity.

This is not an omission but a design choice. By withholding exhaustive disease detail, the theory remains capable of addressing multiple domains without privileging any single pathology without privileging any single pathology [1]. What is retained is not disease identity, but structural logic.

© The Author(s), under exclusive license to Springer Nature Singapore Pte Ltd. 2026

K. Komura, *Adjustment Cord Theory*,
https://doi.org/10.1007/978-981-95-7645-6_8

To bridge this gap between abstract theory and disease-specific elaboration, Adjustment Cord Theory introduces the concept of structural motifs.

8.2 Structural Motifs as Recurrent Patterns of Constraint

A structural motif refers to a recurrent configuration in how tension is constrained, redirected, or forced through specific passages across distinct systems. Motifs are not mechanisms, pathways, or components. They are patterns of necessity that persist despite variation in constituent elements.

Such motifs may manifest as persistent focal constraint despite distributed activity, oscillatory redistribution between competing passages, or apparent stability maintained by reciprocal limitation. These patterns recur across biological scales and disease categories, even when molecular identities differ entirely.

The analytical value of motifs lies in their abstraction. By focusing on how constraint is organized rather than on what constitutes the system, motifs enable comparison without reduction. They capture similarity of structure without implying similarity of cause.

Motifs therefore function as carriers of generality despite variation in constituent elements [2]. They allow insight gained in one context to inform inquiry in another without assuming equivalence at the level of components or mechanisms.

8.3 Why Motifs Are Necessary but Insufficient

While structural motifs provide orientation, they do not constitute explanations or prescriptions. Identifying a motif does not determine where intervention should occur or how it should be executed. Rather, motifs clarify which kinds of interventions are structurally plausible and which are likely to be ineffective or destabilizing.

Motifs therefore function as constraints on reasoning rather than as solutions. They narrow the space of viable hypotheses without dictating specific actions. This role is essential in complex systems, where the number of possible interventions far exceeds the number of structurally coherent ones.

Importantly, motifs do not replace disease-specific analysis. They precede it. Molecular detail, cellular dynamics, and clinical context remain indispensable, but they are approached with structurally informed expectations rather than with unbounded speculation.

In this sense, motifs reduce error before they increase precision.

8.4 Transferability Without Dilution

The strength of Adjustment Cord Theory lies in its capacity to transfer insight without diluting specificity. Structural motifs enable this transfer by preserving relational logic while allowing unrestricted variation at the component level.

Transferability does not imply uniform application. It implies that insights can travel across contexts without collapsing differences. What transfers is not content, but structure.

By maintaining this separation, the theory remains open--ended. Disease-specific elaboration can proceed independently, without threatening the integrity of the framework. Conversely, the framework can evolve without requiring revision of disease-level detail.

This architecture allows Adjustment Cord Theory to function as a durable reference point rather than a transient synthesis.

8.5 Structural Motifs as Entry Points for Future Elaboration

Structural motifs are not endpoints of theory. They are entry points for future elaboration. Once a motif is identified, disease-specific research can explore how particular mechanisms instantiate that structure under given constraints.

Such elaboration may take many forms: molecular studies, computational modeling, clinical stratification, or therapeutic design. Adjustment Cord Theory does not prescribe these directions. It provides a scaffold upon which they can be constructed coherently.

In this way, motifs serve as interfaces between general theory and specialized inquiry. They define where detail becomes meaningful without demanding that it be supplied within the theoretical framework itself.

References

1. Goldenfeld N, Kadanoff LP. Simple lessons from complexity. Science. 1999;284:87–9.
2. West GB, Brown JH, Enquist BJ. A general model for the origin of allometric scaling laws in biology. Science. 1997;276:122–6.

Chapter 9
Methodological Implications

9.1 From Theory to Practice Without Reduction

Adjustment Cord Theory (ACT) does not prescribe specific methods, datasets, or analytical pipelines. Its contribution is methodological in a different sense. It reframes how methods are selected, interpreted, and combined.

Rather than asking which technique is most powerful, ACT asks which techniques are capable of revealing constraint, necessity, and redistribution. Methods are evaluated not by resolution or scale, but by their ability to inform structural inference.

This chapter outlines methodological implications of this stance, focusing on integration rather than replacement.

9.2 Integrating Multi-modal Data Through Structural Questions

Modern biomedical research generates vast amounts of heterogeneous data: transcriptomics, proteomics, imaging, spatial profiling, and longitudinal clinical records. Integration of these modalities is often framed as a technical challenge [1]. From an ACT perspective, it is primarily a conceptual challenge.

© The Author(s), under exclusive license to Springer Nature Singapore Pte Ltd. 2026

K. Komura, *Adjustment Cord Theory*,
https://doi.org/10.1007/978-981-95-7645-6_9

Data modalities should not be integrated because they are available, but because they interrogate different aspects of structure. Each modality captures a projection of the system under specific constraints.

Structural relevance emerges when multiple modalities converge on the same passage-like configuration, especially under perturbation or over time. Such convergence suggests necessity rather than coincidence.

9.3 Longitudinal Observation and Perturbation as Structural Probes

Static snapshots are insufficient for identifying adjustment cords. Structural necessity is revealed through response, not through presence.

Longitudinal observation allows assessment of persistence, adaptation, and phase transition [2]. Perturbation, whether therapeutic or experimental, acts as a probe that exposes which passages cannot be bypassed.

From an ACT standpoint, failure of compensation is more informative than magnitude of change [3]. The focus shifts from how much changes to what cannot remain the same.

9.4 Visualizing Tension, Constraint, and Passage

Visualization plays a central role in ACT, not as illustration but as reasoning aid. Conventional network diagrams emphasize connectivity and density. ACT-oriented visualization prioritizes flow, restriction, and inevitability.

Effective representations may abstract away components in favor of depicting routes, bottlenecks, and redistribution under perturbation. Temporal layering and comparative views across conditions are often more informative than detailed static maps.

Visualization should therefore be evaluated by whether it helps identify unavoidable passages, not by aesthetic completeness.

9.5 From Structural Insight to Hypothesis Generation

ACT does not replace hypothesis-driven research. It reorders it.

Rather than generating hypotheses based on association or prominence, ACT guides hypothesis generation toward passages of necessity. Hypotheses become questions about constraint: What happens if this passage is weakened? What alternatives remain? Does the system reorganize or collapse?

Such questions are fewer but more discriminating. They favor falsifiability over breadth and coherence over coverage.

9.6 Methodology as a Moving Alignment

Finally, ACT treats methodology itself as dynamic. As system configurations change, the relevance of methods shifts. What once revealed constraint may later obscure it.

Methodological rigor therefore requires periodic realignment between question, system state, and analytical tool. No method remains optimal across all phases.

This flexibility is not weakness. It is a recognition that structure, not technique, should anchor inquiry.

References

1. Menche J, et al. Uncovering disease-disease relationships through the incomplete interactome. Science. 2015;347:1257601.
2. Othmer HG. Self-Organization in Nonequilibrium Systems (G. Nicolis and I. Prigogine). SIAM Rev. 1982;24:483–5.
3. Kitano H. Biological robustness. Nat Rev Genet. 2004;5:826–37.

Chapter 10
Designing for Structured Complexity

10.1 What Adjustment Cord Theory Makes Visible

Adjustment Cord Theory does not offer a comprehensive explanation of disease. It makes something else visible: the distinction between what is prominent and what is necessary.

By focusing on constraint, passage, and redistribution, the theory reframes how complex systems are understood. Disease behavior is no longer interpreted as the consequence of dominant components alone, but as the outcome of how tension is forced to move through limited routes imposed by structure.

This shift clarifies why certain interventions fail despite strong rationale, why others succeed unexpectedly, and why adaptation is the rule rather than the exception. What matters is not how strongly a component acts, but how little the system can act without a given passage.

In making this distinction explicit, Adjustment Cord Theory provides a language for reasoning about necessity without reducing complexity to simplicity.

© The Author(s), under exclusive license to Springer Nature Singapore Pte Ltd. 2026

K. Komura, *Adjustment Cord Theory*,
https://doi.org/10.1007/978-981-95-7645-6_10

10.2 What the Theory Deliberately Leaves Unresolved

Adjustment Cord Theory does not claim to identify adjustment cords automatically, universally, or definitively. It does not provide algorithms, thresholds, or fixed procedures. These absences are intentional.

Structural necessity is context-dependent. It emerges under constraint, shifts with configuration, and reveals itself only through interaction with time and perturbation. Any attempt to freeze it into a static rule would contradict its defining properties.

The theory therefore resists closure. It leaves open questions regarding identification, measurement, and intervention, not as weaknesses, but as invitations for further inquiry.

By doing so, it preserves adaptability. The framework remains compatible with evolving data, methods, and domains without requiring revision of its core principles.

10.3 Toward Disease-Specific Elaboration Without Dilution

The value of Adjustment Cord Theory lies not in replacing disease-specific research, but in orienting it. Structural motifs, adjustment cords, and dynamic reconfiguration provide a scaffold upon which detailed pathology can be explored without losing coherence.

Disease-specific elaboration is therefore not a continuation of this book, but a parallel endeavor. Each domain must identify how structural necessity is instantiated within its own constraints.

In this sense, Adjustment Cord Theory does not conclude inquiry. It repositions it. It invites researchers and clinicians to ask not only what changes, but what cannot be bypassed when change occurs.

Designing for structured complexity is not about control.
It is about alignment:

aligning intervention with necessity,
inquiry with constraint,
and explanation with structure.

Afterword

This book does not offer a final answer to complex disease.

It offers a way to see constraint.

Adjustment Cord Theory (ACT) proposes that many failures of intervention arise not from lack of mechanistic detail, but from acting on what is prominent rather than what is necessary. If a disease state can be described as a tension map, then intervention can be redescribed as a problem of structural alignment: where tension is forced to pass and how that passage can be adjusted without creating new obligations.

Across the chapters, three spiral archetypes—convergent, divergent, and drum-type—are used as minimal structural units to describe how phenotypes emerge, fluctuate, and stabilize. Visible phenotypes can be treated as projections of latent tension architectures. In some domains, morphology offers a particularly readable surface—yet the framework is not bound to any organ. The same language can be carried into multi-organ diseases, where tension is distributed across immune circuits, vascular interfaces, stromal remodeling, and behavioral/physiological constraints.

A central implication follows: treatment should be discussed not only by targets and strength but also by *structural depth*—surface adjustment, tension reconfiguration, and nodal intervention. Durable change is expected when intervention touches the adjustment cord itself, shifting trajectories

© The Editor(s) (if applicable) and The Author(s), under exclusive license to Springer Nature Singapore Pte Ltd. 2026
K. Komura, *Adjustment Cord Theory*,
https://doi.org/10.1007/978-981-95-7645-6

and reshaping relapse patterns rather than merely suppressing manifestations.

ACT is not complete without method. Network analysis can outline the static scaffold; temporal multi-omics can reveal migrating centers of tension; and AI-based inference can translate high-dimensional structure into patient-specific hypotheses. In this sense, a disease digital twin is not a futuristic decoration—it is a practical extension of the same structural question: *Where is the adjustable point, and what happens if we touch it?*

If there is one request to the reader, it is this: do not treat ACT as a doctrine. Treat it as an instrument. Use it to redraw familiar problems, to test where the "neck" of the system truly lies, and to remain attentive to paradoxical reactions as structural feedback rather than mere noise.

The value of this theory will be determined not by how elegantly it explains the past, but by whether it helps clinicians and researchers design interventions that make the future trajectory of disease measurably different.

FSC
www.fsc.org

MIX
Papier aus verantwortungsvollen Quellen
Paper from responsible sources
FSC® C105338

If you have any concerns about our products,
you can contact us on
ProductSafety@springernature.com

In case Publisher is established outside the EU,
the EU authorized representative is:
Springer Nature Customer Service Center GmbH
Europaplatz 3, 69115 Heidelberg, Germany

Printed by Libri Plureos GmbH
in Hamburg, Germany